The Ultimate Alkaline Diet Cookbook

The Fastes Alkaline
Guide to Eat well and Reclaim your Health

Cody Read

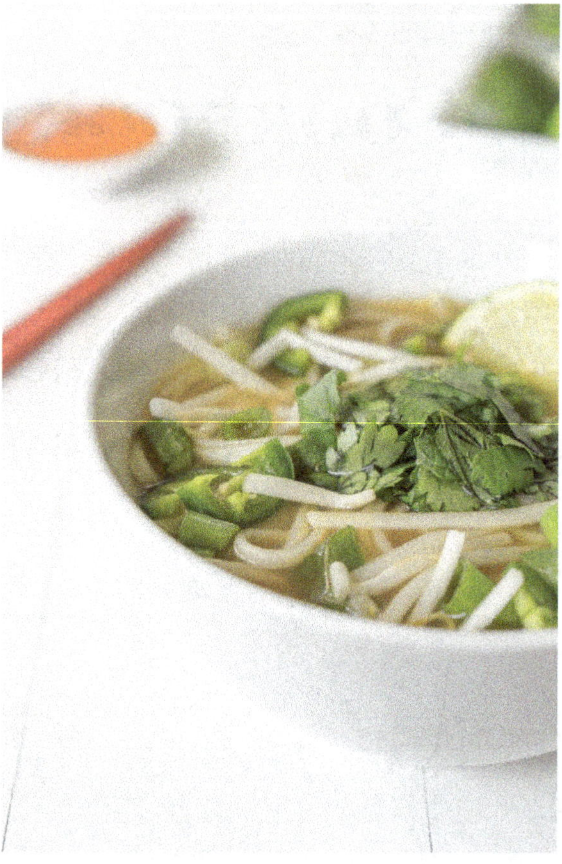

By reading this document, the reader agrees that under no circumstances is the author responsible for any losses, direct or indirect, which are incurred as a result of the use of information contained within this document, including, but not limited to, — errors, omissions, or inaccuracies.

Table of Contents

Greek Vegetable Salad

Servings: 2

Total Time: 15 minutes

Ingredients

- 2 red bell peppers, diced
- 3 large tomatoes, chopped
- 1 bunch kale (about 14 leaves), stems removed and sliced into thin ribbons
- 10 black olives in oil, sliced in half
- 1 red onion, halved and sliced
- 2 celery stalks, diced plus leaves
- 3 radishes, sliced
- ½ cup green or brown lentils, cooked

Dressing

- ½ cup lemon juice
- ¾ cup cold pressed olive oil
- 1 garlic clove, minced
- 1 teaspoon ground oregano
- 1 teaspoon dried basil

- ½ teaspoon ground cumin
- ¼ teaspoon sea salt
- ¼ teaspoon black pepper
- 1 teaspoon flaxseeds

Directions

1. Combine the vegetables, olives & lentils in a bowl and set aside.
2. Place all dressing ingredients in a blender and blend until smooth and creamy.
3. Pour dressing over the vegetable mixture and lightly massage. Let rest at least 15 minutes before serving.

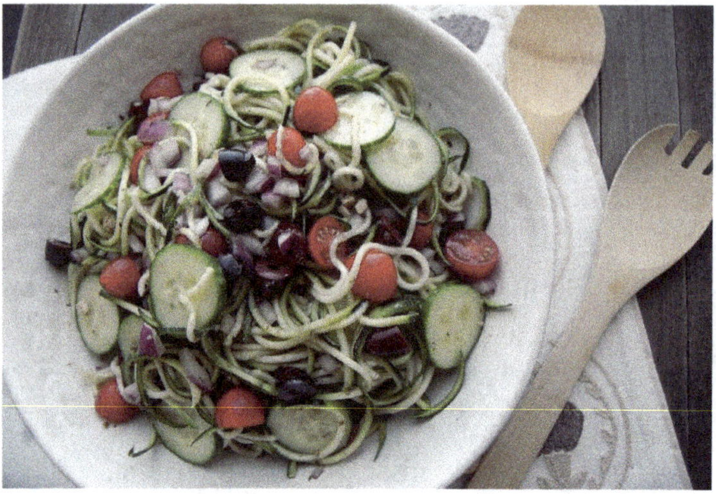

Sweet & Spicy Vegetable Wrap

Servings: 2

Total Time: 30 minutes

Ingredients

- 1 small red beet, peeled and diced small
- 1 small sweet potato, peeled and diced small
- 1 turnip, peeled and diced small
- 2 tablespoons olive oil
- 1 teaspoon Himalayan salt
- 1 teaspoon smoked paprika
- ¼ teaspoon cumin
- 2 sprouted grain tortilla wraps
- ½ cup arugula
- ½ cup sprouts

Dipping Sauce

- ½ cup unsweetened, plain yogurt
- 1 tablespoon lime juice
- 1 teaspoon cumin
- ½ teaspoon Himalayan salt

- ¼ teaspoon black pepper, crushed

Directions

1. In a small bowl, combine dipping sauce ingredients and mix well. Set aside for at least 15 minutes.

2. On a baking tray lined with parchment paper place diced vegetables and drizzle with olive oil. Sprinkle with salt, paprika and cumin. Toss to combine and make sure vegetables are evenly coated. Place in oven at 375°F/190°C and roast 20 minutes.

3. Lay out each tortilla wrap and spread dipping sauce on top followed by the arugula and then the roasted vegetables.

4. Top with sprouts and roll up each wrap. Serve with extra dip on the side.

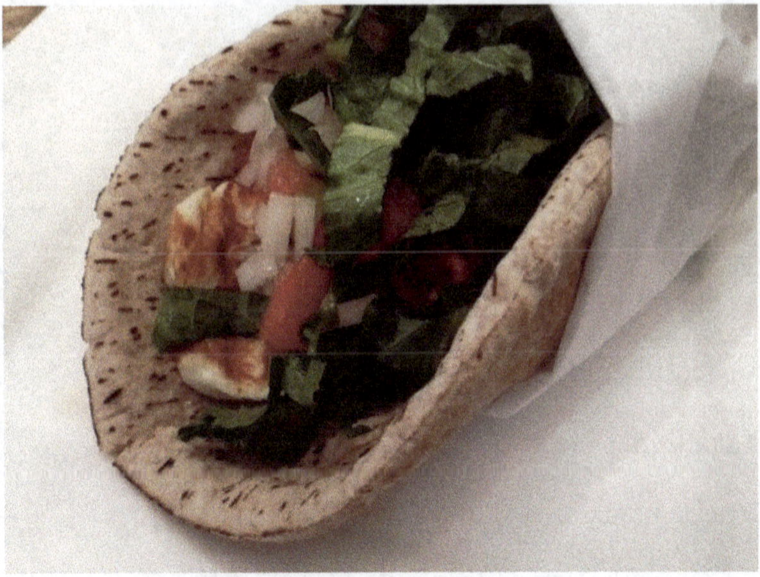

Mediterranean Millet Salad

Servings: 2

Total Time: 30 minutes

Ingredients

- ½ cup millet, rinsed
- 1 cup water
- 12 cherry tomatoes, quartered
- 1 cucumber, diced small
- 1 scallion, sliced
- ½ cup black olives, quartered
- 1 cup parsley, chopped finely
- ¼ cup mint, chopped finely
- 2 tablespoons pine nuts, toasted

Dressing

- ¼ cup extra virgin olive oil
- 1 lemon, juiced
- 1 large garlic clove, minced
- 1 teaspoon dried oregano
- 1 teaspoon dried basil

- ½ teaspoon Himalayan salt

Directions

1. Prepare millet by bringing water to a rolling boil in a saucepan over medium high heat. Stir in millet, reduce heat to low and put lid on the pan. Cook for approximately 20 minutes.

2. Whisk together dressing ingredients and set aside.

3. Combine millet, chopped vegetables, olives, parsley, mint and dressing in a large bowl. Gently toss to combine. Top with pine nuts and parsley for garnish.

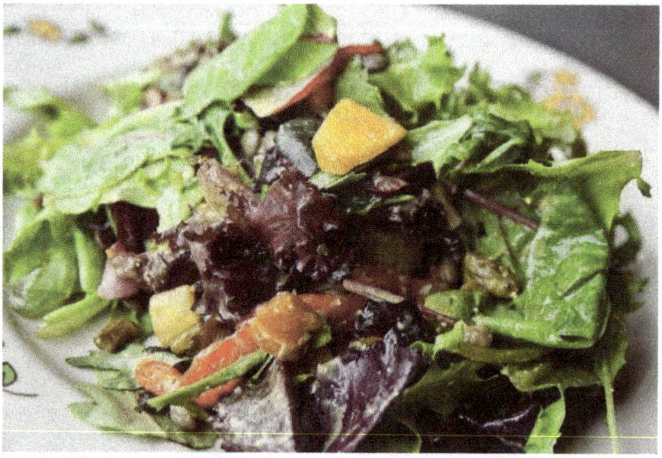

Grab & Go Zucchini Rolls

Servings: 2

Total Time: 20 minutes

Ingredients

- 2 medium zucchinis, sliced very thin lengthwise using vegetable peeler
- 1 carrot, sliced into matchsticks
- 1 cucumber, sliced into matchsticks
- 2 radishes, sliced thinly
- ½ cup red cabbage, shredded
- 1 avocado, peeled and sliced
- 1 small bunch cilantro

Super Greens Hummus

- ½ cup chickpeas, drained and rinsed (or prepared fresh)
- ¼ cup soaked cashews
- 1 tablespoon tahini
- 1 cup kale leaves, de-stemmed and chopped
- ½ cup parsley
- 1 teaspoon of paprika

- 1 garlic clove
- ½ lemon, juiced
- 1/3 cup olive oil
- 1 teaspoon Himalayan salt

Directions

1. Make the Super Greens Hummus by adding all the Super Greens Hummus ingredients to a blender or food processor and blending until creamy and smooth, adding more olive oil if the hummus is too thick.

2. Lay out each of the zucchini ribbons on a flat surface. Spread hummus on each of the zucchini ribbons. On top of the hummus add carrots, cucumber, radish, cabbage, avocado and some of the cilantro.

3. Begin rolling the one side of the zucchini ribbon until reaching the other end.

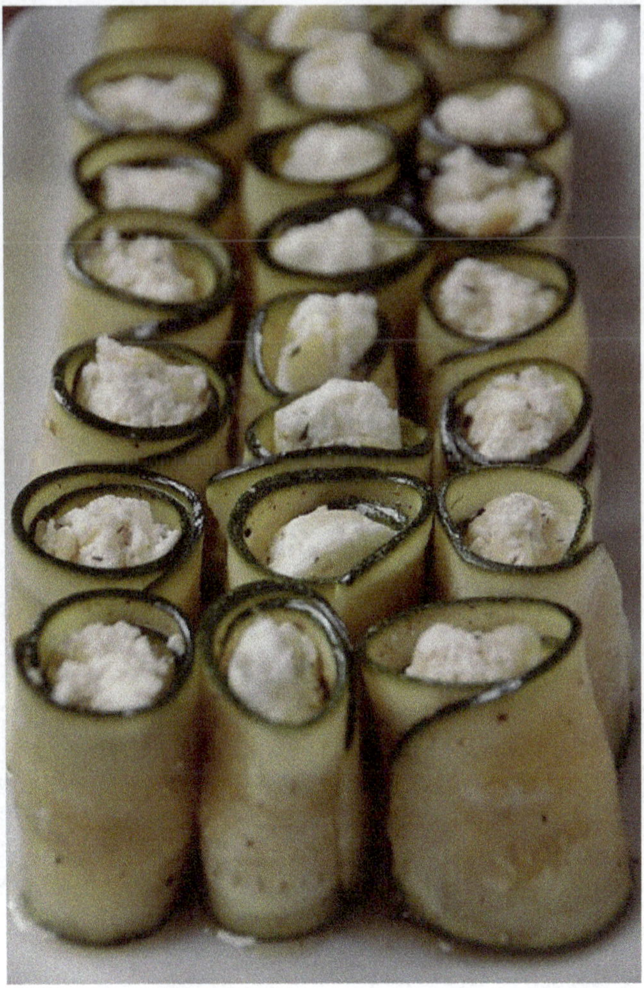

Apple Kale Salad

Servings: 2

Total Time: 5 minutes

Ingredients

- 3 cups kale, stems removed and sliced into thin ribbons
- 1 cucumber, diced
- 1 Granny Smith apple, cored and diced
- ½ cup cooked brown rice
- 1 avocado diced
- ¼ cup pomegranate seeds
- ½ cup walnuts, chopped

Dressing

- ¼ cup apple cider vinegar
- ¼ cup olive oil
- 3 tablespoons lemon juice
- 1 lemon, zested
- 1 teaspoon Himalayan salt
- ½ teaspoon black pepper, crushed

Directions

1. Place kale, cucumber, apple, brown rice, avocado, pomegranate seeds and walnuts in a large bowl.

2. Whisk together dressing ingredients in a separate bowl until well combined.

3. Drizzle dressing over greens and toss to combine.

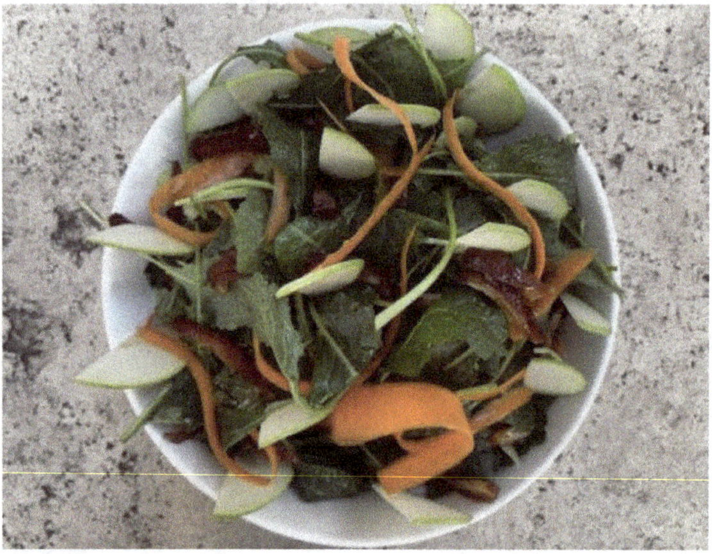

Lentils & Greens Rice Pilaf

Servings: 2

Total Time: 10 minutes

Ingredients

- ¼ cup vegetable broth
- ½ cup pak choi, sliced
- ½ cup broccoli florets
- 1 carrot, diced
- ½ lemon, juiced
- 1 cup of wild rice, cooked
- ½ cup green or brown lentils, cooked
- 1 cup arugula
- 1 teaspoon Himalayan salt
- 1 teaspoon black pepper, crushed
- 1 teaspoon crushed almonds
- 1 avocado

Directions

1. Add vegetable broth to a medium skillet over medium high heat. Let it come to a slight simmer and add pak choi, broccoli, carrot and lemon juice. Cook for 5 minutes.
2. Turn heat off and stir in wild rice, lentils, arugula, salt, pepper and almonds.
3. Transfer to plates and top with avocado slices.

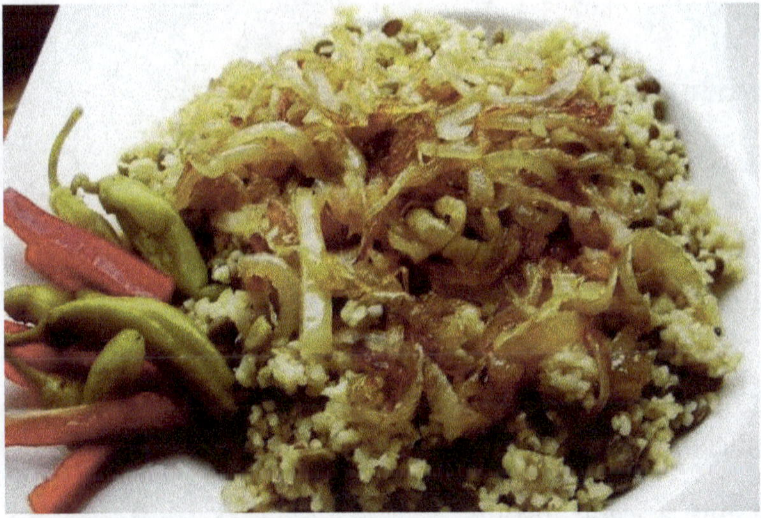

Collard Wraps

Servings: 2

Total Time: 10 minutes

Ingredients

- 2 large collard leaves
- ¼ cup brown rice, cooked
- ¼ cup purple cabbage, shredded
- ¼ cup carrots, shredded
- 1 zucchini, spiralized
- ¼ cup broccoli sprouts

Avocado Spread

- 1 avocado, mashed
- 1 tablespoon ground flaxseeds
- 1 tablespoon chia seed
- 1 teaspoon chili powder
- 1 garlic clove, minced
- ½ lemon, juiced
- 1 teaspoon Himalayan salt
- ½ teaspoon black pepper, crushed

Directions

1. Make avocado spread by adding all the Avocado Spread ingredients to a bowl and combining well.

2. Open up the collard leaves on your work surface making sure each is flat and without many holes.

3. Spread avocado spread evenly over each wrap and top with brown rice. Add vegetables starting with the cabbage and ending with the sprouts.

4. Fold the bottom of the wrap and then fold in each side. Secure with a toothpick and enjoy.

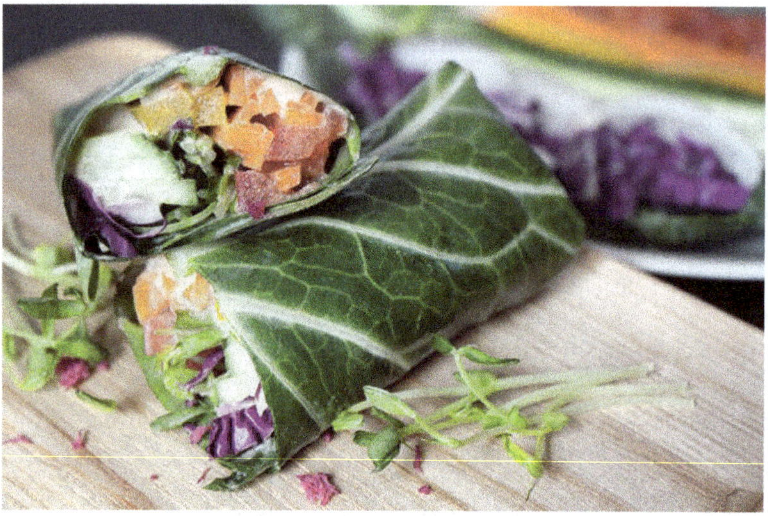

Sesame Greens & Tofu

Servings: 2

Total Time: 15 minutes

Ingredients

- 1 ½ tablespoons toasted sesame oil
- 2 tablespoons olive oil
- 8 ounces extra firm tofu, cubed
- 2 cup broccoli florets, chopped finely
- ½ cup red bell pepper, diced
- 1 garlic clove, minced
- 2 tablespoons soy sauce or tamari
- ½ lemon, juiced
- 1 teaspoon sesame seeds

Directions

1. Heat ½ tablespoon sesame oil and 1 tablespoon olive oil in a pan over medium low heat and add tofu. Cook for 10 minutes, turning occasionally. Set tofu aside and add 1 more tablespoon of olive oil and 1 tablespoon of sesame oil.

2. Stir in broccoli, red bell pepper and garlic. Cook for 5 minutes or until softened. Add tofu back to the pan and stir in soy sauce and lemon juice. Top with sesame seeds and serve.

Roasted Carrot & Quinoa Salad

Servings: 2

Total Time: 25 minutes

Ingredients

- 1 pound carrots, peeled and sliced into 1 inch pieces
- 1 teaspoon coconut oil, melted
- 1 teaspoon smoked paprika
- 1 teaspoon cumin
- 1 teaspoon chili powder
- ¼ teaspoon salt
- 2 cups arugula
- ½ cup quinoa, cooked
- 2 tablespoons pepitas, toasted
- 1 cup broccoli sprouts

Dressing

- 1 garlic clove, minced
- ¼ cup tahini
- 1 lemon, juiced
- 1 teaspoon turmeric

- ¼ teaspoon salt
- ¼ teaspoon black pepper, crushed
- 3 tablespoons water

Directions

1. Preheat oven to 400°F/205°C. Toss carrots with coconut oil, paprika, cumin, chili powder and salt. Layer in an even layer on a baking tray lined with parchment paper. Bake for 20 minutes or until lightly browned, turning once.

2. While carrots are cooking, make dressing by combining all the dressing ingredients in a blender or food processor. Add more water if mixture is too thick.

3. In a large bowl, combine roasted carrots, quinoa, arugula and dressing together.

4. Top with pepitas and sprouts.

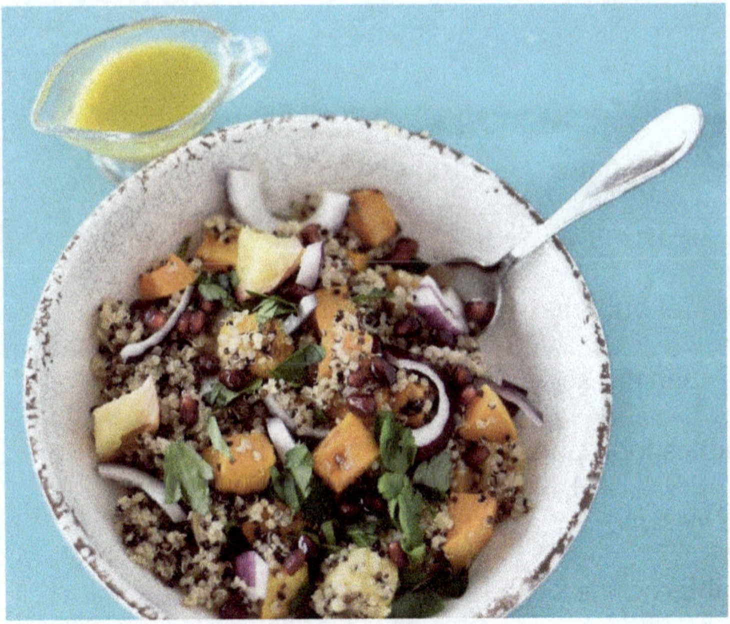

Raw Fennel Salad with Citrus Dressing

Servings: 2

Total Time: 10 minutes

Ingredients

- 1 pomegranate, seeds removed
- 1 cup carrots, grated
- 1 fennel bulb, halved and then sliced
- 1 grapefruit, segmented
- 1 tablespoon pumpkin seeds, toasted

Citrus Dressing

- 3 tablespoons fresh lime juice
- 5 tablespoons fresh orange juice
- 1 tablespoon olive oil
- 1 teaspoon apple cider vinegar
- ½ teaspoon nutmeg
- 1 teaspoon Himalayan salt
- 1 teaspoon black pepper, crushed

Directions

1. In a large bowl, combine Citrus Dressing ingredients and whisk well.

2. Add to the large bowl the pomegranate seeds, carrots, fennel and grapefruit. Toss well to combine and garnish with the pumpkin seeds.

Taco Salad Bowl

Servings: 2

Total Time: 20 minutes

Ingredients

- 2 cups kale, stems removed and sliced into thin ribbons
- 1 tablespoon olive oil
- 1 carrot, shredded
- 5 green onions, sliced
- 1 red bell pepper, sliced into strips
- 1 ½ cups cooked brown lentils
- ½ cup walnuts, toasted
- 1 tablespoon tomato paste
- 1 garlic clove, minced
- ½ teaspoon smoked paprika
- ½ teaspoon chili powder
- ½ teaspoon cumin
- ½ teaspoon Himalayan salt
- ¼ cup water
- ½ avocado, sliced

Cashew Ranch Dressing

- 1 ¼ cup cashews, soaked overnight and drained
- ½ cup water
- 1 lemon, juiced
- 1 teaspoon apple cider vinegar
- ¼ cup parsley
- 3 tablespoons chives, chopped
- 2 tablespoons fresh dill, chopped
- 1 teaspoon nutritional yeast
- 1 teaspoon Himalayan salt
- 1 teaspoon black pepper, crushed

Directions

1. In a large bowl, place kale and drizzle with olive oil. Massage kale gently and set aside for 5 minutes before adding in the carrots, green onions and red bell pepper.

2. In a food processor add brown lentils, walnuts, tomato paste, garlic, smoked paprika, chili powder, cumin, salt and water to make taco "meat". Pulse together until crumbly.

3. Clean food processor and add ingredients for the Cashew Ranch Dressing. Process until smooth.

4. Place lentil & walnut “meat” on top of the vegetables, top with avocado slices and drizzle with Cashew Ranch dressing.

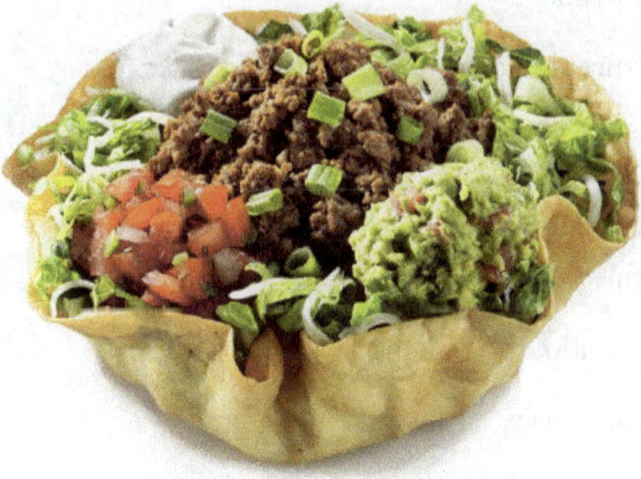

Veggie & Mango Sushi

Servings: 2 (1 sushi roll per serving)

Total Time: 35 minutes

Ingredients

- 2 nori sheets
- ½ zucchini, cut into thin strips
- 1 carrot, cut into thin strips
- 1 cup mango, cut into thin strips
- 1 cup sprouts
- 1 avocado, sliced

Cauliflower Rice

- ½ head cauliflower, cut into florets
- ½ tablespoon olive oil
- ½ cup quinoa, cooked and warmed
- ½ teaspoon tamari
- ½ teaspoon apple cider vinegar
- ½ teaspoon coconut aminos
- 1 teaspoon sesame seeds

Directions

1. Process cauliflower florets in a food processor until a rice consistency is formed. Place cauliflower rice on a parchment paper lined baking tray, drizzle with olive oil and roast in an oven that has been preheated to 425°F/220°C for 25 minutes.

2. Place roasted cauliflower and warm quinoa in a large bowl and add tamari, vinegar, coconut aminos and sesame seeds. Combine well until it becomes sticky and holds together slightly when pushed together.

3. On a bamboo mat or tea towel in front of you, place a nori sheet and add half of the cauliflower rice at the end closest to you but leaving a slight space.

4. Place half of the zucchini, carrot, mango, sprouts and avocado on top of the rice. Roll up starting with the edge closest to you and pressing in as you go.

5. Repeat with the remaining nori, cauliflower rice and vegetables/fruit.

6. Slice each roll into 8 pieces and serve.

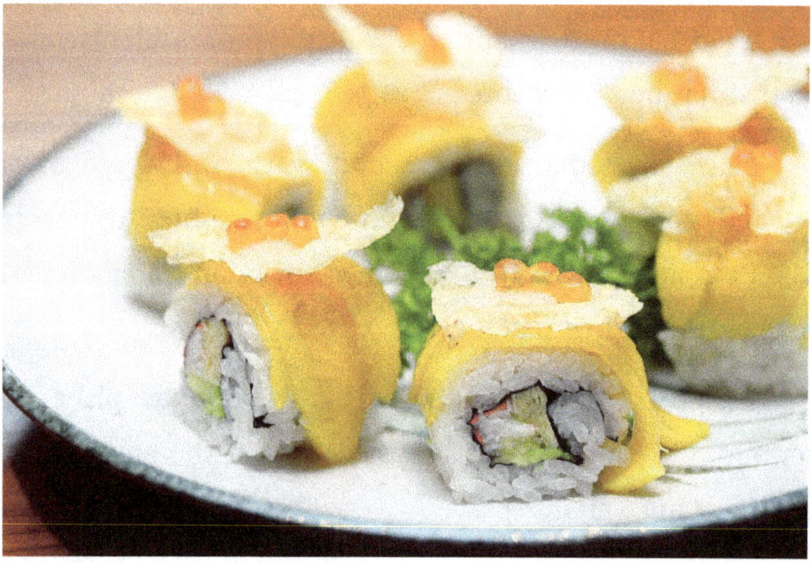

Buddha Bowl

Servings: 2

Total Time: 35 minutes plus 5 hours in the fridge

Ingredients

- 1 bunch kale, stems removed and sliced into thin ribbons
- 1 tablespoon olive oil
- 1 teaspoon lemon juice
- 2 cups quinoa, cooked
- 1 cup lentils, cooked
- 10 cherry tomatoes, halved
- 1 zucchini, made into noodles with a spiralizer
- 1 avocado, sliced
- 1 tablespoon black sesame seeds
- 1 tablespoon green onions, thinly sliced

Tahini Dressing

- ¼ cup tahini
- ¼ cup warm water
- 1 teaspoon lemon juice
- 1 tablespoon maple syrup

- ½ teaspoon turmeric
- 1 garlic clove, minced

Pickled Radishes

- 3 red radishes, thinly sliced
- ¼ cup apple cider vinegar
- ¼ cup water
- 1 tablespoon honey
- 1 teaspoon Himalayan salt
- ½ jalapeno, seeded and diced
- 1 teaspoon whole black peppercorns

Directions

1. In a jar that has a lid, place in all Pickled Radishes ingredients. Mix well and let sit for 5 hours in the fridge with the lid on. Make sure the radishes are always covered with liquid.

2. Prepare Tahini Dressing by place all the ingredients in a small bowl and whisk together until smooth. If mixture is too thick, thin it out with more water.

3. Place kale in a large mixing bowl and massage gently with the olive oil and lemon juice. Let rest 10 minutes.

4. To assemble and serve, place kale at the bottom of a bowl and top with quinoa, lentils, tomatoes, zucchini noodles, avocado and pickled radishes. Drizzle with Tahini Dressing and sprinkle with black sesame seeds and green onions.

Sweet Roasted Chickpeas

Servings: 2

Total Time: 35 minutes

Ingredients

- 2 cups chickpeas, cooked
- 1 tablespoon coconut oil
- 1 teaspoon cinnamon
- 1 teaspoon nutmeg
- 1 teaspoon coconut sugar

Directions

1. Preheat oven to 400°F/205°C. Toss chickpeas with coconut oil in a small oven proof bowl. Bake in the oven for 30 minutes, mixing frequently.
2. While chickpeas bake, add cinnamon, nutmeg and sugar to a separate medium sized bowl.
3. Remove chickpeas from oven and place immediately in the bowl with the spices. Toss well to coat.
4. Lay on a plate and let cool before serving.

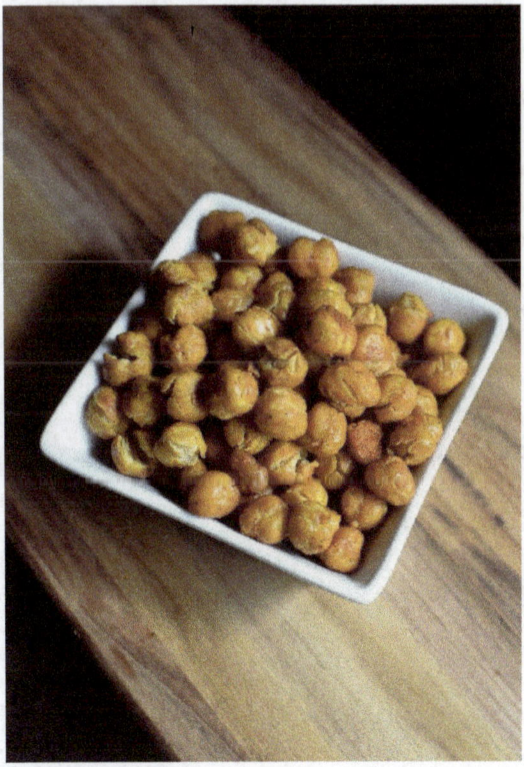

Roasted Broccoli with Tahini Dip

Servings: 2

Total Time: 35 minutes

Ingredients

- 2 cups broccoli, cut into large florets
- 2 tablespoons olive oil
- ½ teaspoon Himalayan salt
- ¼ teaspoon turmeric
- 2 tablespoons tahini
- 1 tablespoon warm water
- ½ tablespoon honey

Directions

1. Preheat oven to 400°F/205°C. Toss broccoli with oil, salt and turmeric in a small oven proof bowl. Bake in the oven for 30 minutes, turning once.

2. While broccoli roasts, whisk together the tahini, water, and honey in a small bowl.

3. Remove broccoli from oven and serve immediately with the tahini dip.

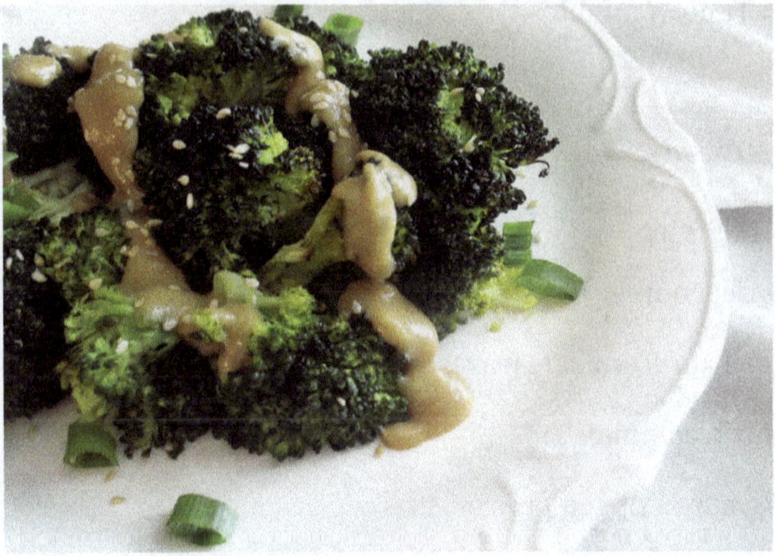

Green Goddess Smoothie

Servings: 1

Total Time: 5 minutes

Ingredients

- 1 avocado
- ½ cucumber
- 1 cup of fresh kale leaves, stems removed
- 1 peeled lime
- ½ cup chopped parsley
- 1 cup water

Directions

1. Place all ingredients into a high speed blender. Pulse a few times to get started then mix on high until smooth.

Spicy & Smooth Green Shake

Servings: 2

Total Time: 5 minutes

Ingredients

- 1 cucumber
- 2 tomatoes
- 1 avocado
- 1 cup spinach leaves
- 1 lime, juiced
- ½ jalapeno, seeded
- ¼ teaspoon red pepper flakes
- ½ cup water
- 1 teaspoon spirulina powder

Directions

1. Combine all ingredients in a blender and combine until smooth. Add more if too thick.

Tropical Smoothie

Servings: 2

Total Time: 5 minutes

Ingredients

- 1 cup pineapple, diced
- 1 cup watermelon, diced
- 2 limes, juiced
- ½ cup cauliflower florets, steamed
- ½ cup cilantro, chopped
- ½ cup coconut water

Directions

1. Place all ingredients in a blender and blend until smooth.

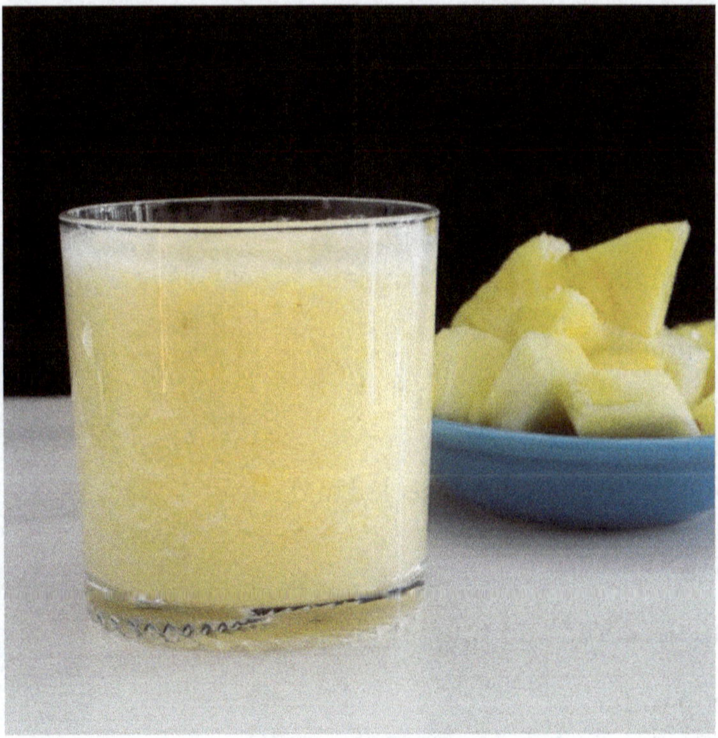

Ginger Blast Smoothie

Servings: 2

Total Time: 5 minutes

Ingredients

- 2 cucumbers, roughly chopped
- 1 lemon, juiced
- 1 lime, juiced
- 2 inch piece of ginger, peeled and sliced
- 2 cups spinach
- 1 apple, cored and roughly chopped
- 1 cup water
- 2 teaspoons chia seeds

Directions

1. Place all ingredients except the chia seeds in a blender and blend until smooth. Stir in chia seeds and serve.

Spicy Golden Tea

Servings: 2

Total Time: 10 minutes

Ingredients

- 16 ounces water
- 1 inch of fresh turmeric root, peeled and diced small
- 1 inch of fresh ginger root, peeled and diced small
- 2 lemon slices (do not boil, add to tea before serving)
- 2 teaspoons raw honey
- Pinch black pepper

Directions

1. Place water, turmeric and ginger in a small saucepan and bring to a boil over medium heat.
2. Reduce heat and let simmer another 5 minutes.
3. Pour into glasses and add lemon slices, honey and pepper before serving.

Lemon Basil Zinger

Servings: 2

Total Time: 5 minutes

Ingredients

- 2 small lemons, peeled and seeds removed
- 1 ½ tablespoons of coconut oil
- ½ green apple, cored and chopped
- 3 ½ cups water
- ½ teaspoon Himalayan salt
- 1 teaspoon raw honey
- 3 fresh basil leaves
- 4 - 5 ice cubes
- 2 lemon slices

Directions

1. Place all ingredients in a blender except the lemon slices and blend until fully combined.
2. Serve with a fresh lemon slice.

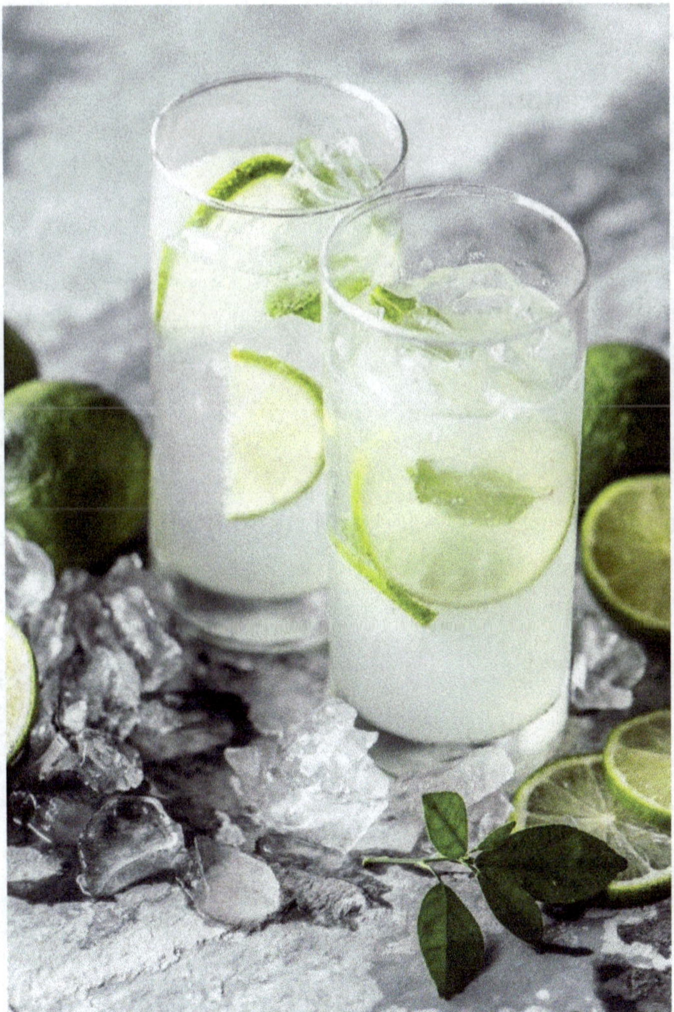

Bloody Mary Shake

Servings: 2

Total Time: 10 minutes

Ingredients

- 1 small cucumber
- 1 celery stalk
- 3 tomatoes
- ½ red bell pepper, seeded and roughly chopped
- 1 garlic clove
- 1 lemon, juiced
- ½ jalapeno, seeded
- ¼ teaspoon pepper
- ½ teaspoon tamari sauce
- ¼ teaspoon cayenne pepper
- 6 - 8 ice cubes
- 4 olives

Directions

1. Place all ingredients in a blender except for the olives and blend until fully combined.

2. Garnish with olives and serve.

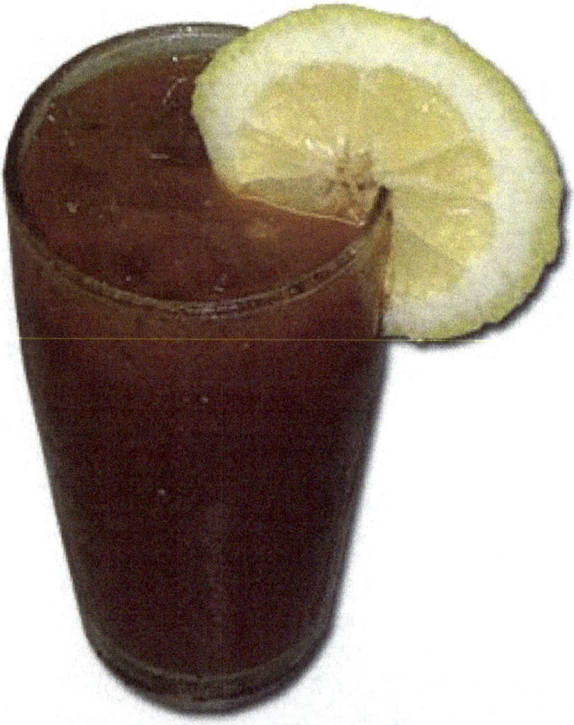

Alkaline Veggie Juice

Servings: 2

Total Time: 5 minutes

Ingredients

- 2 carrots
- 1 cucumber
- ¼ head green cabbage
- 1 cup kale
- ½ lemon
- ½ cup parsley
- 1 inch piece ginger
- 1 inch piece turmeric

Directions

1. Place all ingredients in a juicer and serve immediately.

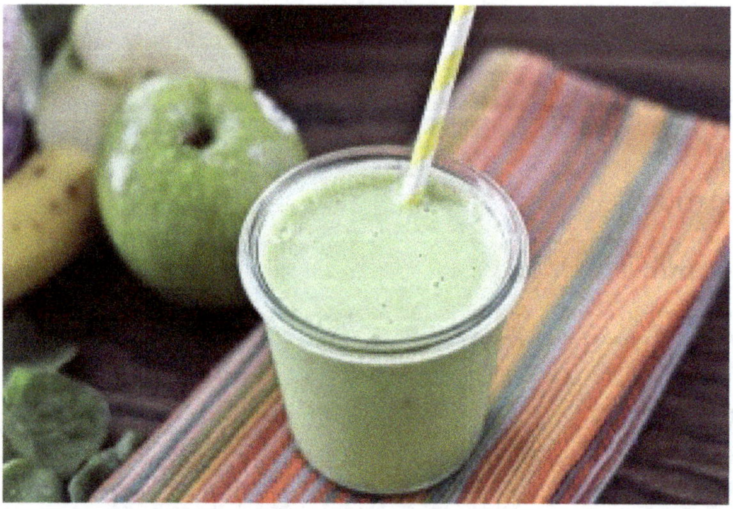

Coconut Lime Smoothie

Servings: 1

Total Time: 5 minutes

Ingredients

- 4 ounces fresh coconut meat
- ½ cup coconut water
- ½ cup coconut milk
- 1 tablespoon coconut oil
- 1 lime, peeled
- 1 banana, frozen
- 3 - 4 ice cubes
- ½ teaspoon lime zest

Directions

1. Place all ingredients except the lime zest in a blender and blend on high until fully combined.

2. Garnish with lime zest and serve.

Berry Blast Smoothie

Servings: 1

Total Time: 5 minutes

Ingredients

- 1 cup spinach
- ¼ cup blueberries
- ¼ cup raspberries
- 1 tablespoon raw cashew butter
- 1 tablespoon ground flaxseed
- 1 tablespoon coconut oil
- 1 cup almond milk
- 1 tablespoon chia seeds
- 1 tablespoon hemp hearts

Directions

1. Place all ingredients except the chia seeds and hemp hearts in a blender and combine.
2. Stir in chia and hemp hearts and serve.

Minty Morning Shake

Servings: 2

Total Time: 5 minutes

Ingredients

- ¾ cup unsweetened coconut milk
- ¼ cup canned coconut milk
- 1 cup fresh spinach
- ½ avocado
- ½ cup fresh mint leaves
- 2 bananas, frozen
- 2 dates, pitted
- 1 teaspoon vanilla extract
- ¼ teaspoon Himalayan salt
- ¼ teaspoon peppermint extract
- 6 - 8 ice cubes
- 1 teaspoon cacao nibs
- 2 fresh mint leaves

Directions

1. Place all ingredients except the cacao nibs and 2 fresh mint leaves in a blender until smooth.

2. Garnish with cacao nibs and mint leaves before serving.

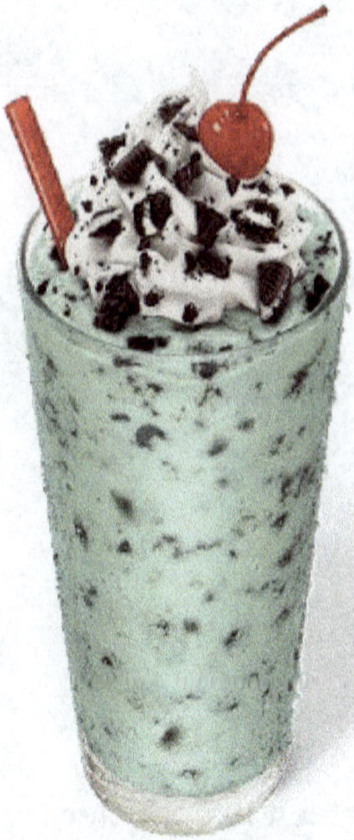

Green Tea & Fruit Smoothie

Servings: 2

Total Time: 5 minutes

Ingredients

- 2 ripe mangoes, peeled and chopped
- ½ cup raspberries
- ¼ cup pineapple, diced
- 1 ripe frozen banana, peeled
- 1 cup unsweetened almond milk
- 1 lime, juiced
- 2 teaspoons matcha green tea powder
- 3 - 4 ice cubes

Directions

1. In a blender combine all ingredients until smooth and serve.

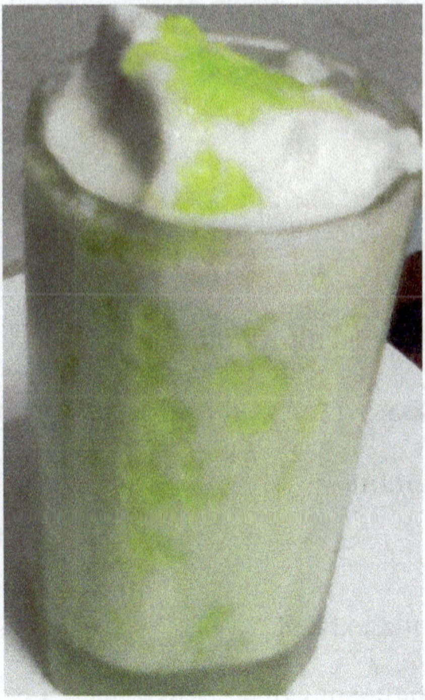

Apple Pie Smoothie

Servings: 2

Total Time: 5 minutes

Ingredients

- 1 red apple, cored and chopped
- ½ frozen banana
- 1 ½ cups unsweetened almond milk
- 3 dates, pitted, soaked for 15 minutes and drained
- 1 teaspoon cinnamon
- ½ teaspoon nutmeg
- ½ teaspoon vanilla extract
- ¼ teaspoon Himalayan salt

Directions

1. In a blender combine all ingredients until smooth and serve.

Morning Alkaline Lemon Water

Servings: 1

Total Time: 2 minutes

Ingredients

- 8 ounces of alkaline water, either lukewarm or slightly warmed (not boiling)
- ½ lemon, juiced

Directions

1. In a cup mix together the water and lemon juice.
2. Serve immediately either first thing upon waking (before consuming breakfast or other beverages) or before a meal.

Detox Juice

Servings: 1

Total Time: 5 minutes

Ingredients

- 2 small beets, peeled
- 1 carrot, peeled
- 1 small apple
- 1 lemon, peeled and seeds removed
- 1 ½ inch piece of ginger

Directions

1. Place all ingredients in your juicer and serve immediately.

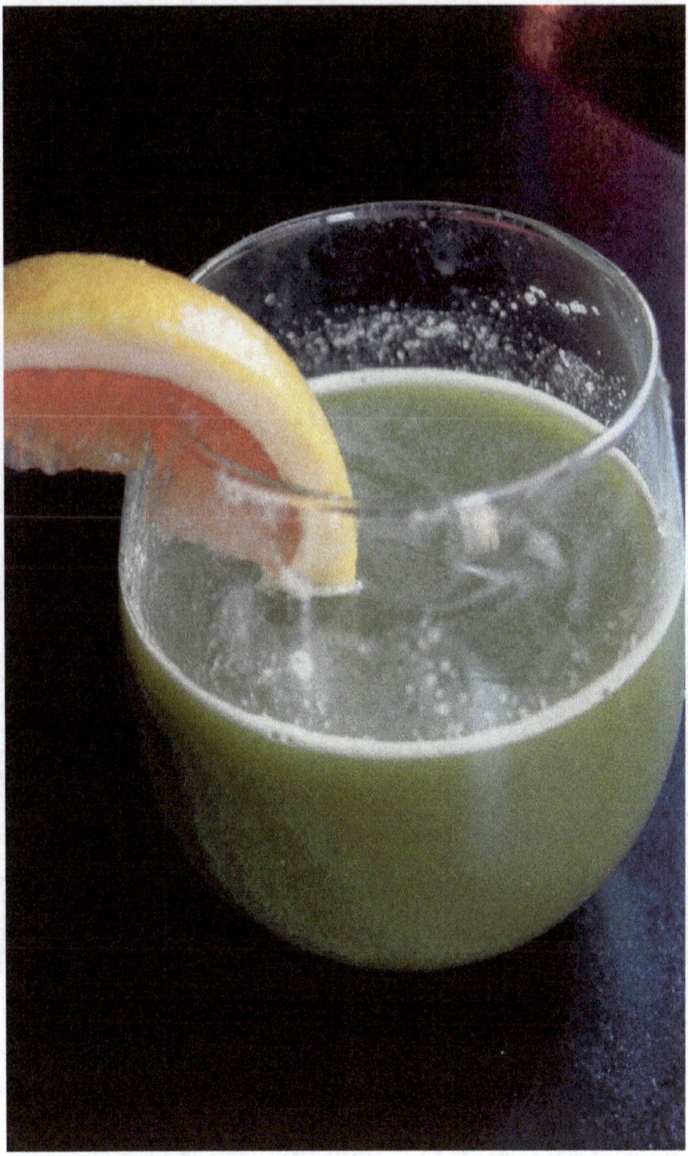

Fruity Summer Lemonade

Servings: 2

Total Time: 2 minutes

Ingredients

- 3 lemons
- 1 apple
- 1 ½ cups water
- 1 cup fresh strawberries, washed and hulled
- 1 cup watermelon, cubed
- ½ cup mint
- 1 teaspoon raw honey
- 5-6 ice cubes

Directions

1. Juice lemons in a juicer and set aside the juice.
2. Juice apples in a juicer and combine juice with lemon juice in a blender.
3. Add water, strawberries, watermelon, mint, honey and ice cubes to the blender and blend until smooth.

4. Serve immediately.

All Day Detox Water

Servings: 2

Total Time: 2 minutes

Ingredients

- 16 ounces water
- 6 lemon slices
- 10 cucumber slices
- ¼ teaspoon Himalayan salt
- 5 - 6 ice cubes (optional)

Directions

1. In a small pitcher, combine water, lemon, cucumber, salt and ice cubes (if using).

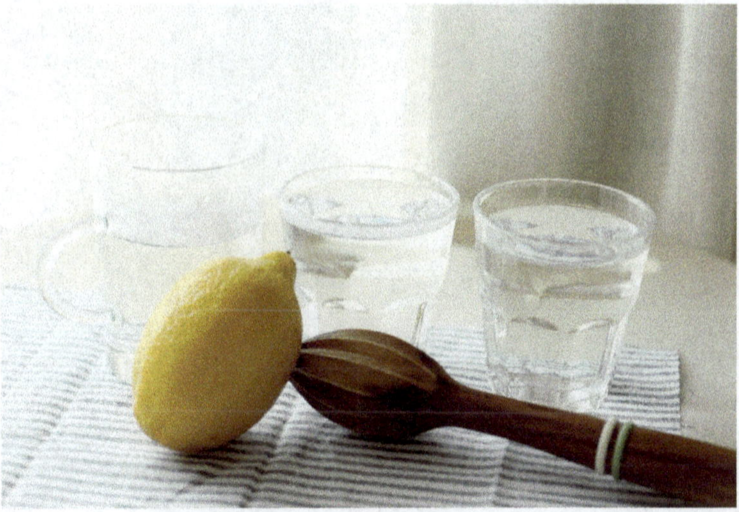

Watermelon Mint Water

Servings: 2

Total Time: 2 minutes

Ingredients

- 16 ounces water
- ½ cup watermelon, cubed
- 8 mint leaves, torn
- ¼ teaspoon Himalayan salt
- 5 - 6 ice cubes (optional)

Directions

1. In a small bowl, using the back end of a spoon, muddle together the watermelon, mint and salt.

2. Add watermelon mint mixture to a pitcher and fill with water and ice cubes (if using).

Glow Juice

Servings: 2

Total Time: 5 minutes

Ingredients

- 2 green apples
- 1 cup collard greens, chopped
- 1 cup parsley
- ½ large cucumber
- 1 inch piece of ginger

Directions

1. Place all ingredients in juicer. Serve juice immediately.

Creamy Green Smoothie

Servings: 1

Total Time: 5 minutes

Ingredients

- ½ cucumber
- 2 cups kale, stems removed
- ½ cup frozen broccoli
- ½ avocado
- 2 ounces silken tofu
- 1 inch ginger, grated
- 1 large lime, juiced
- ¼ teaspoon cayenne pepper
- ½ cup ice
- ½ cup unsweetened coconut milk

Directions

1. Place all ingredients in blender and blend until smooth. Serve immediately.

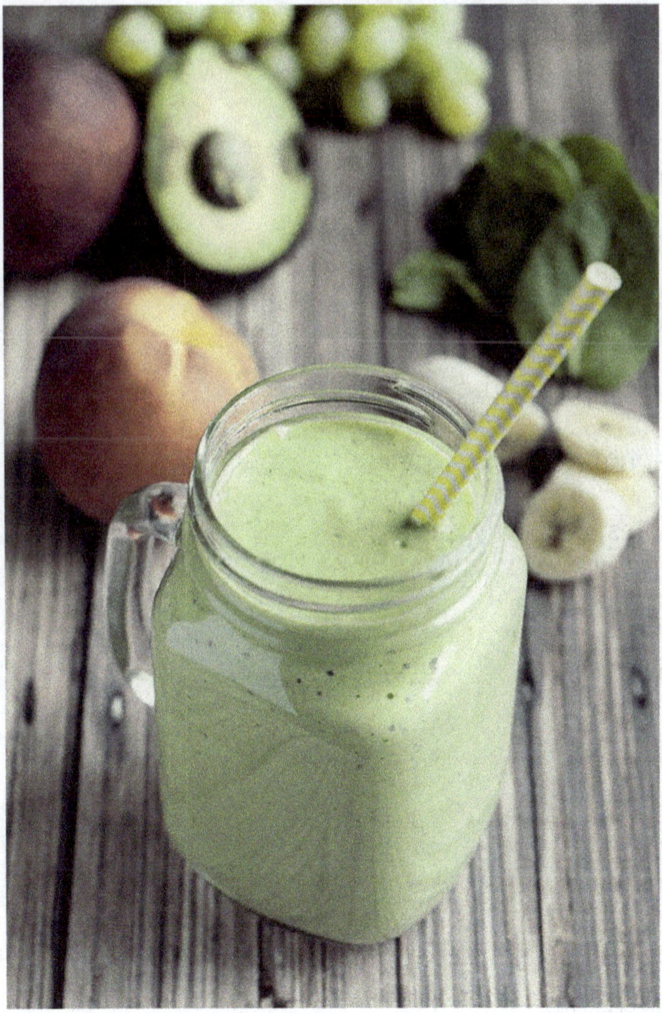

Creamy Orange Smoothie

Servings: 1

Total Time: 5 minutes

Ingredients

- 3 medium oranges, peeled
- ½ banana, frozen
- ½ cup almond milk
- ½ teaspoon vanilla extract
- 1 ½ tablespoons raw honey
- 1 cup spinach
- ½ lime, juiced
- 2 cups ice cubes

Directions

1. Place all ingredients in a high speed blender and combine. Serve immediately.

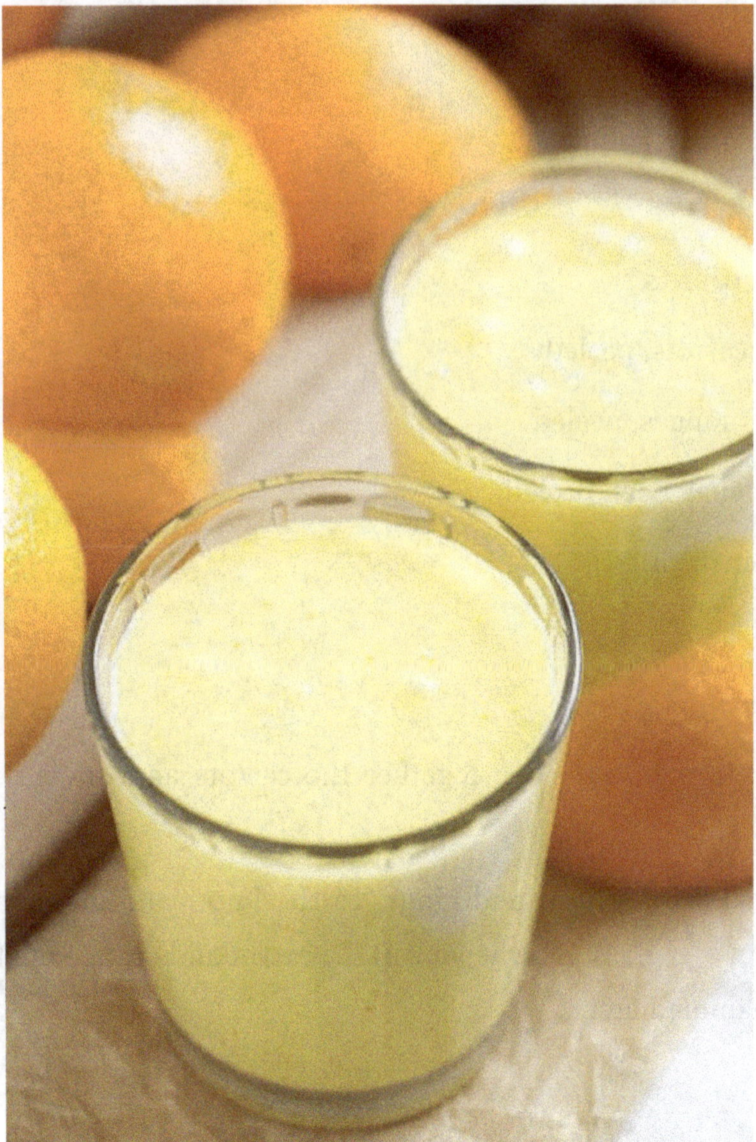

Sunrise Juice

Servings: 1

Total Time: 5 minutes

Ingredients

- 2 carrots, peeled
- 2 oranges, peeled
- 1 small beet, peeled
- 1 inch ginger

Directions

1. In a juicer, juice together the carrots and oranges. Set aside.

2. Juice the beet and ginger in the juicer and place at the bottom of a glass. Slowly pour in the carrot and orange mixture. Serve immediately.

Mulled Cider

Servings: 2

Total Time: 5 minutes

Ingredients

- 1 apple seeded, cored and quartered
- 1 tablespoon raw honey
- ¼ orange peel with pith
- 1 inch piece ginger, grated
- ¼ teaspoon ground cinnamon
- Pinch of ground cloves
- Pinch of allspice
- Pinch of Himalayan salt
- 2 cups warm water

Directions

1. Combine all ingredients in a high speed blender. Serve warm.

Melon Melody

Servings: 2

Total Time: 5 minutes

Ingredients

- 1 cup honeydew melon, cubed
- 1 cup watermelon, cubed
- 1 cup cantaloupe, cubed
- 3 - 4 mint leaves

Directions

1. In a high speed blender, place all ingredients and combine until smooth.

Mango Colada

Servings: 2

Total Time: 5 minutes

Ingredients

- 1 cup frozen mango, cubed
- ½ banana, frozen
- 1 cup pineapple
- 1/2 cup unsweetened almond milk
- 1 can unsweetened coconut milk
- ½ lime, juiced
- 5 - 6 ice cubes

Directions

1. In a high speed blender, place all ingredients and combine until smooth.

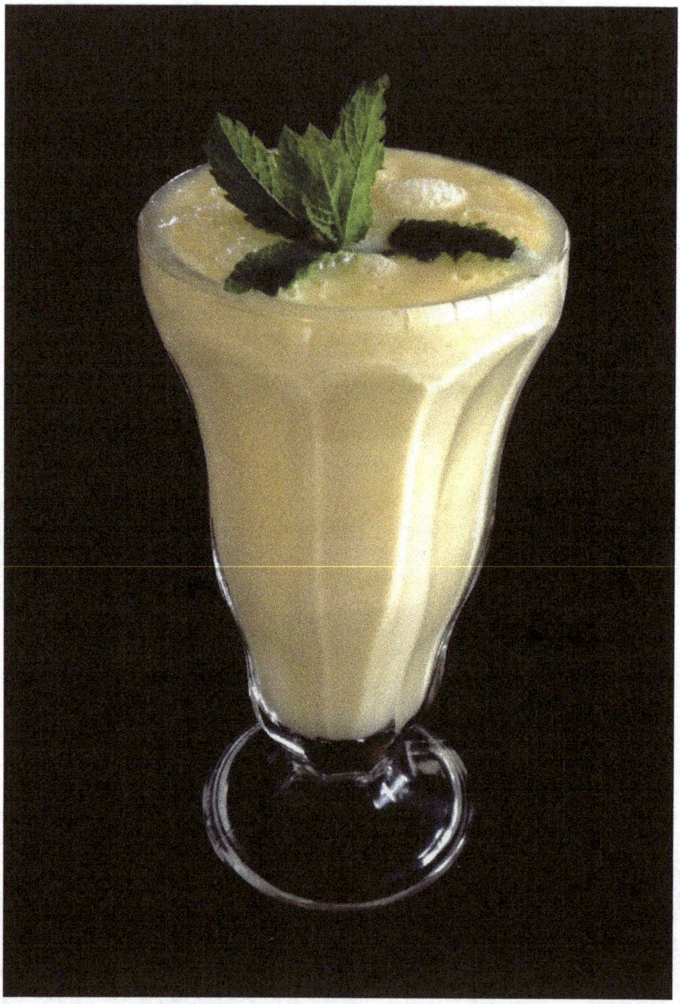

Herbal Tonic

Servings: 2

Total Time: 10 minutes

Ingredients

- 34 ounces water
- 1 lemon, peel grated and then juiced
- 2 teaspoons fresh thyme leaves
- 2 teaspoons fresh sage leaves
- 1 teaspoon rosemary leaves
- 2 inch piece ginger root, grated
- 1 inch piece turmeric root, grated
- 2 teaspoons apple cider vinegar
- 2 teaspoons raw honey

Directions

1. In a small saucepan over medium heat, bring the water to a boil.

2. Add in lemon peel, lemon juice, thyme leaves, sage, rosemary, ginger, turmeric and vinegar. Simmer for 3 - 4 minutes.

3. Strain liquid into two mugs and stir a teaspoon of honey into each before serving.

Probiotic Citrus Drink

Servings: 2

Total Time: 5 minutes

Ingredients

- 2 large grapefruits, juiced
- 4 lemons, juiced
- 10 ounces water
- 1 teaspoon of acidophilus
- 1 clove of fresh garlic, grated
- 2 inches of fresh root ginger, grated
- 1 tablespoon olive oil
- 1 teaspoon matcha powder

Directions

1. Add all ingredients to a blender and combine. Serve immediately.

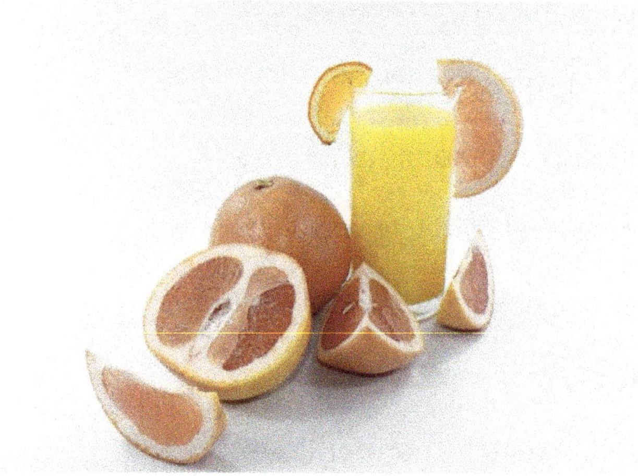

Acid Buster Juice

Servings: 2

Total Time: 5 minutes

Ingredients

- 3 large kale leaves
- 2 celery stalks (and leaves)
- 1 cucumber
- 1 cup arugula
- ½ cup parsley
- ½ inch of fresh root ginger
- ½ lemon
- 8 ounces water
- 2 teaspoons apple cider vinegar

Directions

1. Juice all ingredients in a juicer.

Detox Stimulator Juice

Servings: 2

Total Time: 5 minutes

Ingredients

- 1 cucumber
- 1 bunch kale
- 2 cups watercress
- 1 lemon
- 1 lime
- ½ grapefruit
- ½ inch ginger
- 1 small beetroot
- 1 small carrot

Directions

1. Juice all ingredients in a juicer. Add up to ½ cup water if juice is too thick.

Carrot Dream Smoothie

Servings: 1

Total Time: 5 minutes

Ingredients

- 1 cup unsweetened almond milk
- 1 tablespoon almond butter
- ½ banana, frozen
- ½ inch fresh ginger, grated
- 1 teaspoon cinnamon
- ¼ teaspoon nutmeg
- 3 carrots, shredded
- 1 tablespoon chia seeds
- 1 teaspoon raisins

Directions

1. Blend all ingredients except the chia seeds and raisins in a high speed blender until smooth and combined.
2. Stir in the chia seeds and garnish with raisins.

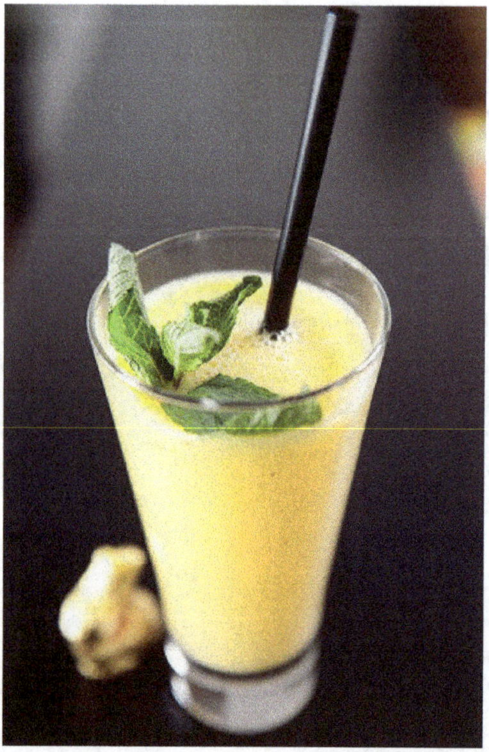

Southwest Stuffed Sweet Potatoes

Servings: 2

Total Time: 1 hour

Ingredients

- 2 sweet potatoes
- 2 tablespoons of coconut oil
- ½ cup black beans, rinsed and drained
- 1 shallot, sliced
- 3 cups spinach
- Pinch of dried red chili flakes
- Pinch of cumin
- 1 avocado, peeled and sliced

Dressing

- 3 tablespoons olive oil
- 1 lime, juiced
- 1 teaspoon cumin
- Handful of cilantro, minced
- Salt and pepper

Directions

1. Preheat oven to 400°F/205°C. Clean sweet potatoes and pierce several times with a fork. Place sweet potatoes on a baking tray lined with parchment paper and bake approximately 50 minutes or until soft.

2. Allow 5 minutes for sweet potatoes to cool.

3. While sweet potatoes are cooling heat skillet over medium heat and add coconut oil, shallot and black beans. Cook for 5 minutes then add spinach, dried chili flakes and cumin. Cook an additional 1 minute.

4. In a small bowl whisk together dressing ingredients.

5. Slice sweet potatoes down the middle and stuff with black bean mixture. Top with avocado slices.

6. Drizzle dressing over the sweet potatoes and serve.

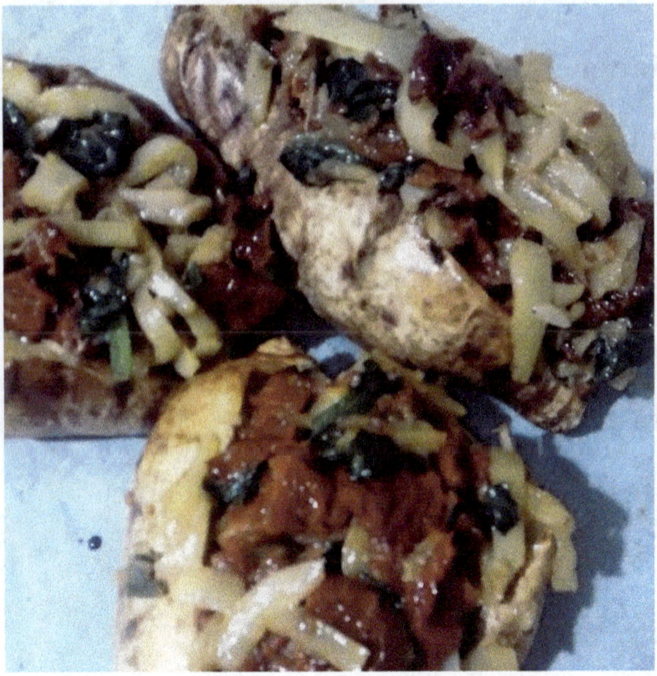

Coconut Cauliflower with Herbs & Spices

Servings: 2

Total Time: 30 minutes

Ingredients

- ¼ cup coconut oil, melted
- ½ tablespoon ground cumin
- ¼ teaspoon ground coriander
- 1 teaspoon ground turmeric
- ¼ teaspoon black pepper, ground
- 1 large cauliflower, chopped into small florets
- 2 tablespoons pine nuts, toasted
- 1 tablespoon cilantro, minced
- ½ tablespoon mint, chopped roughly
- 1 tablespoon raisins
- Himalayan salt

Directions

1. Preheat oven to 425°F/220°C. In a large bowl, mix together coconut oil, cumin, coriander, turmeric and black pepper. Fold in cauliflower and toss until well coated.

2. Spread cauliflower on baking tray and place in the oven for 20 minutes. Remove from oven and transfer to serving bowl.

3. Mix pine nuts, cilantro, mint, raisins and salt with the cauliflower and serve warm.

Zoodles with Avocado Cream Sauce

Servings: 2

Total Time: 15 minutes

Ingredients

- 1 tablespoon coconut oil
- 1 zucchini, spiralized
- 1 avocado, pitted and flesh removed
- 2 tablespoons olive oil
- ½ lemon, juiced
- 1 tablespoon water
- 2 tablespoons cilantro, minced and divided
- 1 teaspoon Himalayan salt
- ½ teaspoon black pepper, ground
- 2 tablespoons pepitas, toasted

Directions

1. Melt coconut oil in a medium skillet over medium-high heat. Add zucchini noodles and cook 3-5 minutes. Turn off heat.

2. In a blender, combine the avocado, olive oil, lemon juice, water, 1 tablespoon cilantro, salt and pepper. Mix until well combined and creamy. If too thick, thin out with a little more water.

3. Add sauce to skillet with the zucchini noodles and toss to combine. If serving warm, turn heat to low and heat gently for 2 minutes.

4. Transfer to serving bowl and sprinkle with toasted pepitas and 1 tablespoon cilantro.

Rainbow Pad Thai

Servings: 2

Total Time: 10 minutes

Ingredients

- 3 medium zucchinis, spiralized
- 2 large carrots, shredded
- 3 scallions (green onions), sliced using green parts
- 1 cup red cabbage, shredded
- 1 cup broccoli, finely chopped
- 1 cup daikon radish (or other mostly white radish), shredded
- 1 cup of fresh cilantro, chopped
- 1 avocado, diced

Dressing

- 1 lime, juiced
- ¼ cup tahini
- 1 teaspoon sesame oil
- 1 garlic clove, minced
- 1 teaspoon ginger, minced

Directions

1. Add first seven ingredients for salad into a large bowl and toss to combine.

2. Prepare dressing by whisking together all dressing ingredients until well combined and creamy.

3. Top vegetables with diced avocado and drizzle with dressing.

Creamy Broccoli Slaw

Servings: 2

Total Time: 15 minutes

Ingredients

- 1 head of broccoli
- ¼ cup raisins
- ¼ cup walnuts, chopped
- Pinch of salt
- Pinch of pepper

Dressing

- 3 tablespoons water
- 2 teaspoons cumin
- 2 teaspoons coriander
- 1 teaspoon turmeric
- ½ teaspoon ground mustard
- ¼ teaspoon ginger
- 1 tablespoon coconut oil
- 1 tablespoon lemon juice
- 1 tablespoon tahini

Directions

1. Trim broccoli and chop into small florets. Set aside in a large bowl.

2. Prepare dressing by placing all dressing ingredients in a blender and blending until smooth and creamy.

3. Add raisins, walnuts, salt and pepper to broccoli and pour dressing over. Combine until all the broccoli mixture is evenly covered.

CPSIA information can be obtained
at www.ICGtesting.com
Printed in the USA
BVHW061956150621
609639BV00002B/349

9 781803 173627